An Index to the Big Book by Subjects and Steps

"I came to A.A. in order to stop drinking; what I received in return was my life." AA Big Book

"Never be too hard on the man who can't give up drink. It's as hard to give up the drink as it is to raise the dead to life again. But both are possible and even easy for Our Lord. We have only to depend on him." – Matt Talbot

<u>**Sections:**</u>

Index by Subject   **page 9-38**

Index by the 12 Steps   **page 41-48**

Big Book Index
by Subject

Big Book Index by Subject

Subject	Page	P'graph
4th Dimension	8	3
5 types of alcoholics	xxx	3
12 Steps	59	3
18 failed methods to stop drinking	31	3
90 meetings in 90 days	525	4
AA		
for people who want, don't need it	315	4
is home	346	3
meetings- common ground	17	2
meetings- tolerance	19	5
way of life	275	2
Abnormal becomes normal	xxviii	5
Acceptance	417	2
Not expectations	420	4
Act and react	293	3
Actor analogy	60	5
Admit our wrongs honestly	67	3
Adultery	81	2

Alcohol

Avoiding	101	4
Being around it after recovery		
	100	5
	101	1
Can't escape	101	2
Cause of unhappiness	281	
Don't hate it	103	2
Gives you two problems	246	1
Immune through service	89	1
In your home	102	4
Interest in it stops	84	4
Makes you miserable	302	1
Medical effects	140	3
Must be conquered first	98	1
No respecter of status	348	2
Part of every disaster	486	2
Powerless over it	195	2
Recoil from	84	4
Symptom	64	1

Alcoholics

    1 year test   34   2

    Afraid others thought he was insane   195   4

    All I could do was work and drink   363   2

    Always an alcoholic   85   2

    Behavior   141   1

    Best drinker, then drunkest   222   2

    Blackouts   225   2

    283   2

    Brains says I'm an alcoholic   538   2

    Can be professionally successful   39   3

    Can stop for a while   34   2

    Cannot fight alcohol   298   3

    Can't be persuaded   90   1

    Can't leave alcohol alone   34   3

    Can't tell them what to do   224   2

(Alcoholics)

Carry the message	89	1
Change goal to meet behavior	423	4
Chronic slipper	455	3
Crazy things they think	321	1
Definition	44	1
Destructive behavior	21	3
Double life	73	2
Drunkenness can last a long time	291	3
Egocentric	61	3
Excuses	23	2
Experiences of wives	105	2
Everyone knows your secret	351	2
Feeling doomed	7	4
Forgot who I was	487	4
Frequent quitters	152	1
Hangovers	172	4
Happy to possible have brain tumor	412	1
Helping other alcoholics	xvi	2

(Alcoholics)

Hoping for surge	269	4
Hopeless cases (Dr. Jung)	26	4
How to approach one	90	4
Huge ability to drink	173	2
Husband	108	3
I'll do anything	214	9
"Just have a couple"	41	2
Like a tornado	82	4
Like a two-sided coin	382	1
Little thought of consequences	37	4
Men of genius	2	1
Negative personality change	351	1
No cure	33	2
No defense against the first drink	41	3
No motivation can make you quit	195	2
Oblivious that drinking was cause of misery	449	2

(Alcoholics)

Outside view of 139 3

Powerless over alcohol 195 2

Propelled toward destruction
268 1

Practicing one has no rights
549 2

Run to extremes 125 4

Real (alcoholics) 21 2

Sacrifice career for alcohol
361 1

Self-centered/ Selfish 61 3

62 3

Sick 7 2

7 4

90 1

Terrifying to live 518 3

Tragic truth about 23 4

Three types 20 4

Unable to stop 39 2

Unusual behavior 138 2

View of themselves 139 3

Why they drink 22 3

(Alcoholics)

    Withdrawal from others   151   2

    Without defense against first drink

        24   2

    Women alcoholics   33   4

Alcoholic life

    Abnormal   xxviii   5

    Destructive behavior   21   3

    Feeling doomed   7   4

    Jay walking analogy   37   5

    Selfish   7   2

    Tried everything   269   6

Alcoholic thinking   35   2

    175   4

    Booze was the answer   486   1

    Get sober to drink   314   2

    Not as bad as others   40   3

    Only drink to get drunk   184   1

Alcoholic to alcoholic   180   3

Alcoholism

    Allergy and obsession   261   2

    Cancer example   18   1

    Diagnosis   31   4

(Alcoholism)

      Disease- not a moral issue 416 3

      Distorts reality 108 2

      Hits family with no warning 446 1

      Is a blessing 492 3

      Physical symptoms 472 3

      Pitiful, incomprehensible demoralization 488 3

      Relief it is a disease 205 3

      Seems normal xxviii 5

      Shouldn't be kept a secret 115 2

Alimony 79 3

Allergy and obsessions (alcoholism) 261 2

Always an alcoholic 33 2

Amazed before we are halfway through 84 4

Amends

      Are about your own faults 78 1

      Behavior convinces when words don't 83 2

      Dr. Bob making amends 156 2

      Reactions are 90% positive 78 2

(Amends)

To friends <u>and</u> enemies	77	2
Anger, cannot live with it	206	2
Ask God for help	76	2
Be quiet and thank God	75	4
Beer experiment	177	4
Behavior convinces when words don't	83	2
Best to meet God alone	63	3
Big Book- spiritual and moral	45	3
Black eyes	533	2
Blackouts	41	2
	225	2
"Satisfactorily" blacked out	283	2
Lying to achieve	283	2
Small price to pay	321	1
Unpredictable	270	2
Blaming others	66	1
Blinding white flash	405	3
Bottles- only a symbol	103	4

Bottoming out 43 2

xxix 2

Brain says I'm an alcoholic 538 2

Brain tumor, happy I might have one

412 1

Broken promises 177 3

Cancer example 18 1

284 1

Can't leave alcohol alone 34 3

Can't skip Step 5 72 2

Carrying the message to others 89 1

Cease fighting 84 4

Change- miracle 85 1

Change- nothing changed, but everything did

251 2

Childhood- result of how I reacted to my

544 3

Children- alcohol effects upon 106 4

Chronic slipper 455 3

Cleaning out the garbage 559 2

Coin, 2-sided 382 1

Common ground for alcoholics 17 2

Common peril for alcoholics 17 2

Confronting an alcoholic 147 4

Connections, making	216	3
Consequences, little thought of	37	4
Cooperate- never criticize	89	3
Counseling	133	3
Crimes	78	4
Criticism- excuse to drink	555	3
Cure- <u>not</u> cured	85	2
Daily prayer	85	2
Daily reprieve	85	2
Daily walk	101	2
Death- drinking to	557	1
Death- to drink is to die	66	2
Decisions- Relax, don't struggle	86	4
Defenseless vs first drink	41	3
Destroying hope	5	6
Destruction- propelled to	268	1
Destructive behavior	21	3
Devil may care chap (type 4)	159	3
Diagnosis for alcoholism	31	4
Disaster- alcohol was part of every	486	2
Disease- alcoholism is allergy and obsession	261	2
Disease, not a moral issue	416	3

Disease, relief that alcoholism is   205   3
Divine help   43   3
Do the right thing   79   2
Doctor Bob   155   2
                                     171

Don't waste time before doing Step 5
                                     74   3
Double life   73   2
Dr. Jung   26   4
Drinking
        is to die (poison)   66   3
        all you dared in a bar   179   3
        awful ache is gone   276   3
        best drinker, then drunkest 222   2
        Interest in stops   84   4
        How some relate to others   471   1
        No motivation can make you quit
                                     195   2
        No pleasure, dulled pain   204   1
        Powerless over alcohol   195   2
        Relief I don't have to drink
                                     354   4
        Stop to heal liver, then restart
                                     556   4

(Drinking)
    Symptom of deeper trouble 544 1
    To death 557 2
    To go to sleep 296 1
    When the wife is out 176 2
Drugs and booze 423 3
Eating sweets 133 4
Erectile disfunction 134 2
Electricity analogy 48 3
Embedded idea of God 55 3
Emptiness, trying to fill 339 2
Epiphany- I don't have to drink 450 2
Every day in AA for 6 months 474 1
Excuses for drinking 23 2
    37 3
    383 3
Excuses for drinking- criticism 555 3
Eyes 9 2
Failure of will power xxxi 3
Failure, predicting 138 3
Faith without works 14 6
Family- can learn from AA principles 130 3

Family- everyone is ill   122   3

Fear   67   4

     Don't want to live, afraid to die   352   5

     Speaking of it takes away power   218   2

Feelings of doom   7   4

Fighting, stop   103   4

Firing alcoholic employee, may be blessing   141   2

First step- not drinking   122   3

Focus on problem, problem increases   419   3

Focus on the answer, not the problem   417   1

Forgot who I was   487   4

Four horsemen of alcoholism   151   2

Freedom for self-will, pray for   87   2

Friends- don't ask them to stop drinking   102   2

Friends- don't withdraw from   102   3

Gates of death   xxvii   7

Getting well- 2 steps   98   3

Go to any lengths   76   3

God   43   4

        After Step 5, be quiet and thank God
                                       75   4

        Alone judges sexual situation
                                       69   5

        Depend on him, not others 98   2

        Disciplines us   88   3

        Discloses himself to us   57   4

        Divine help   43   3

        Dr. Bob attended church as a child
                                      172   3

        Electricity analogy   48   3

        Every person has embedded idea of
                                       55   3

        If you can't let go, ask him for help 76
        1

        In charge of results, motives don't matter
                                      519   3

        Need God's help   62   3

        Own concept of God   12   3

                                       47   1

        Spirituality is personal decision
                                       50   2

        Meeting alone   63   3

Hangovers- none   172   4
Happy destiny, trudging road of   500   1
Help   xvi   1
Help, outside (counseling)   133   3
Helping others   89   1
                                                   191   3
    Why   193   1
Hemorrhages   557   3
Higher Power   43   4
    God discloses himself to us
                                                   57   4
    Need God's help   62   3
    Ask God for help   76   1
    Best to meet God alone   63   3
    Depend on God, not on others
                                                   98   2
    Divine help   43   3
    Electricity analogy   48   3
    One question   47   2
    Own concept   12   3
                                                   46   3
    Power of the group   229   2
    Spirituality is personal   50   2

Honesty

    Admit our wrongs   67   3

    Must be honest with ourselves   58   1

Hopeless- Dr. Jung   26   4

Housekeeping   73   1

    64   2

Human resources won't work   45   1

Humility- continue, improve, practice   511   2

Husbands

    Types   108   6

    Alcoholism should not be a secret   115   2

    How to treat alcoholic husband   108   3

    Leaving alcoholic husband   111   1

    Nagging   111   2

    135   2

    Unreformable?   111   3

I'm not as bad as you   40   3

Illuminate every dark cranny   75   3

Immune from alcohol in service   89   1

Implicating others   80   1

Insanity 195 4

Interventions 90 4

Inventory

      Big chunks of truth 71 1

      Honest one took 22 months

      468 2

Isolation 370 5

Jaywalking analogy 37 5

Jealousy of AA- wives 119 2

Job loss 116 2

Jumping off point 491 2

Jung 26 4

Just have a couple 41 2

Laughter at AA 132 3

Liquor, interest in stops 84 4

Liquor, recoil from 84 4

Live free of pain and degradation 451 3

Live in the answer, not the problem 417 1

Live without waiting to get drunk 549 4

Liver- stopped to heal, then restarted

556 4

Loneliness- isolation 370 5

Lonely- don't need to be anymore 365 2

Loss- every one replaced with rewards

                                             529   2

Lucid interval   90   2

Man in the bed (story)   157   2

Marriage- both people knew alcoholic couldn't stop

                                             239   3

Marriage

        How to treat alcoholic husband

                                           108   3

        Living hell for a wife   248   3

        To an alcoholic   107   3

Martyr- don't be one   79   3

Medical effects of alcoholics   140   3

Meditation and prayer   85   4

Meeting God alone   63   3

Meetings

        90 in 90 days   525   4

        Can't just sit there   498   3

        Relieve pain   485   3

        Suit up and show up   529   6

Men of genius   2   1

Mending relationships   82   3

Miracle of change   85   1

Moment of clarity   42   3

Moment of grace- action	517	1
Money	78	3
	106	1
Morality	44	4
Morals won't save you	44	4
Morning prayer	86	3
Motives don't matter	519	3
Nagging	111	2
	135	2
Newcomers	181	3
Newcomers- small things make a big difference		
	519	1
Nightly prayer	86	2
Nightmares of the past	73	3
No situation too difficult	104	4
Normies (non-alcoholics)	39	2
Change behaviors to meet goals		
	423	4
hinking onne day I could drink again		
	33	2
One question (higher power)	47	2
One-year test	34	2
Own concept of God	12	3

Personality-negative change from alcohol
                        351   1

Phobia of sleeplessness   177   3

Pills   176   1

        410   2

Pink cloud   304   2

Pitiful, incomprehensible, demoralization
        488   3

Pity- self   269   3

        351   1

Plans   86   3

Plans- out of   517   4

Potential- is a curse   513   2

Powerless over alcohol   195   2

Prayer

        And meditation   85   4

        For patience, tolerance   83   1

        Not selfishly   87   2

        Of surrender   215   5

        Step 3   63   2

        Step 7   76   2

        Thy will be done   88   1

        Try   251   1

(Prayer)

    With wives   87   3

Predicting failure   138   2

Problems

    Don't focus on   419   3

    Alcohol gives you two   246   1

    Continue after drinking stops   117   2

    Of our own making   103   4

    Solved by spiritual principles   42   3

Providence- when the time is right   264   3

Quit for yourself   112   4

Quit one thing at a time   190   2

Quitting- no motivation can make you   195   2

Rebirth   63   1

Recovery   xvii   1

    Two steps   98   3

    Awful ache is gone   276   3

    Going to meetings to relieve pain   485   3

    In AA every day for 6 months   475   2

(Recovery)

In Business	140	2
Problems continue	117	2
Rebirth	63	1
Relief I don't have to drink	354	4
Solution	25	2
The way here could not be an easier path	475	2
Two alternatives	25	4
Will power	40	3
Relapse	120	2
	5	5
Don't try to shield alcoholic after	120	4
One day I could drink again	33	2
Relationships after recovery	99	3
Religious ideation	128	2
Resentment- fatal	66	2
Restoration	558	3
Retirement	32	3
Rights- practicing alcoholic has none	549	2

Rules around drinking	400	1
Sanity returns	84	4
Scylla and Charybdis	175	1
Secret- everyone knows yours	351	2
Self-knowledge is foolishness	40	1
Self-pity	269	3
	351	1
Self-centered/ Selfish	62	3
Foolish and sick	7	2
Think about others	199	2
Self-sufficiency	545	3
Self-will, prayer for freedom from	87	2
Sensitive to criticism	555	3
Serenity- matching calamity	68	3
Service		
4 reasons	181	1
A privilege	274	3
Faith without works is dead		
	14	6
Helping others	89	1
	191	3
Immune from alcohol	89	1
Why help others	193	1
Sex	69	

Shoes	532	2
Simple, not always easy	199	3
Skeletons in the closet	125	2
Skepticism from others	83	2
Sleep- drinking to go to sleep	296	1
	408	4
	177	3
Sobriety		
Trying	312	3
First step is not drinking	122	3
AA teaches us how to handle		
	553	1
	558	4
Awful ache is gone	276	3
Become aware of things around you		
	450	4
Can't do it alone	358	4
Dealing with	559	2
Every loss replaced with rewards		
	529	2
Live a life of its own	451	1
Live without waiting to get drunk		
	549	4
Need fellow alcoholics to stay		
	230	1

(Sobriety)

  Not not drinking, but staying sober   558   5

  Priority   357   2

  Problems continue   117   2

  Relief I don't have to drink   354   4

  Short term   270   1

Solution   25   2

Sorry, don't say   83   1

Soul- be able to call mine my own   273   1

Speaking of fear takes the power away   218   2

Spiritual basis or else   44   3

Spiritual epiphany   373   4

Spiritual experience will conquer   44   1

Spirituality

  Best to meet God alone   63   3

  Can solve all problems   42   3

  Dr. B forced to attend church as child   172   3

  Keep in fit condition   85   1

  Not a theory   83   2

  Personal decision   50   2

Relapse causes	120	2
Religious ideation	128	2
Will conquer	44	1
Importance	35	4
Need God's help	62	3
Those who wronged us are ill	66	5
Spouse in Step 12	90	2
State-this one doesn't work either	514	4
Step 3 Actor analogy	60	4
Step 4	64	3
Step 4 is strenuous	64	3
Step 4 model	64	3
Step 5	72	1
Step 6	76	1
Step 7	76	2
Step 7 prayer	76	3
Step 8/9	76	3
Step 9 instructions	77	3
Step 10	84	3
Step 11	85	4
Step 12	89	1
Step 12- approach spouse	90	2
Steps- original 6	263	1

Stop drinking- bad methods	31	3
Stop drinking- temporarily	34	2
Stories- stick to your own	125	3
Strenuous work	xvii	1
Successful and hopeless	xxv	3
Successful but an alcoholic	39	3
Suicide- afraid to die	352	5
Suicide attempts	488	2
Suicide, too cowardly for it	213	4
Suit up and show up	529	5
Surgery- hoping for	269	4
Surrender	300	1
Survive- how I did it	202	4
Temptation- don't to try shield alcoholic	120	4
Terrifying to live as a drunk	518	3
Thinking about others	199	2
Time travel	41	2
Tolerance in AA	19	5
Tragic truth	23	5
Trivial excuses for drinking	37	3
Trudging the road of happy destiny	500	1
"Trying" to stay sober	312	3
Twelve steps	59	3

Two alternatives 25 4

Types of drinkers 20 3

Types of alcoholics xxx 3

Unable to stop 39 2

Undisciplined 88 2

Vodka- like teleportation 370 3

Ways to stop drinking (that don't work)
31 3

Why alcoholics drink xxxvi 2

22 3

xxvi 2

Will power xxxi 3

40 3

Withdrawal tendency of alcoholics 151 3

Without defense against the first drink
24 2

Wives- jealous of AA 119 2

Women- may drink less 33 4

Work and drink 363 2

Work- confronting and alcoholic 147 4

Work- every organization has alcoholics
149 2

Work- firing an alcoholic may help them
141 2

Work- sacrificing career for alcohol

361   1

Big Book Index
of the 12 Steps

Big Book Index of the 12 Steps

Step	Subject	Page	P'graph
Step 1	Description	59	3
	Newcomers	181	3
Step 2	Description	59	3
Step 3	Description	59	3
	Actor analogy	60	4
	Alcoholism- Symptom	64	1
	Alcoholics- Egocentric	61	3
	Alcoholics-Selfish	61	3
	Best to meet God alone	63	3
	God- need God's help	62	3
	God- best to meet alone	63	3
	Higher power- need God's help	62	3
	Higher power- meet God alone	63	3

(Step 3)

Housekeeping- personal   63   4

Meeting God alone
        63   3

Prayer for Step 3   63   2

Rebirth   63   1

Recovery- rebirth 63   1

Self Centeredness
        62   3

Step 4   Description   59   3

Strenuous   64   3

Admit wrongs honestly
        67   3

Blaming others   66   1

Death- to drink is to die
        66   3

Fear   67   4

Sexual Situation   69   5

Honestly admit wrongs
        67   3

Inventory- Big chunks of truth
        71   1

Inventory- example
        468   2

(Step 4)

    Resentment is fatal   66   2

        Serenity matching calamity
           68   3

        Sex   69

        Spirituality- those who wronged us
        are ill   66   5

        Step 4- usually done more than
        once   72   2

Step 5   Description   59   3

        Step 5 detail   72   2

        Alcoholics- double life
           73   2

        Be quiet and thank God
           75   4

        Can't skip Step 5
           72   2

        Don't waste time before Step 5
           75   1

        Double life   73   2

        Housekeeping   73   1

        Illuminate every dark cranny
           75   3

        Nightmares of the past
           73   3

Step 6   Description   59   3

Step 6- detail   76   1

Ask God for help 76   1

Step 7   Description   59   3

Step 7- detail   76   2

Prayer for Step 7

    76   3

Step 8/9   Step 8-Description

    59   3

Go to any lengths 76   3

Steps 8/9 detail   76   3

Step 9   Description   59   3

Step 9 instructions

    77   3

Adultery   81   2

Alcoholics- like a tornado

    82   4

Alimony   79   3

Amazed before we're halfway
through   83   4

Amends- Dr. Bob

    156   2

Amends is about you

    78   1

Amends- reactions to

    78   2

(Step 9)

Behavior- convince when words don't 83 2

Crimes 78 4

Do the right thing 79 2

Implicating others 80 1

Martyr- don't be one 79 3

Mending relationships 82 3

Money 78 3

Morning prayer 83 1

Prayer for patience 83 1

Skepticism from others 83 2

Sorry- don't say it 83 1

Spirituality- not a theory 83 2

Step 10 Description 59 3

Step 10- details 84 3

Alcohol- interest in it stops 84 4

(Step 10)

Alcohol- will reoil from
84   4

Alcoholics- always alcoholics
85   2

Cease fighting   84   4

Change- miracle 85   1

Cure-not cured   85   2

Daily Prayer   85   2

Daily reprieve   85   2

Drinking- interest stops
85   4

Miracle of change
85   1

Not fighting   85   1

Sanity returns   84   4

Spirituality- keep in fit condition
85   1

Step 11   Description   59   3

Step 11 details   85   4

Decisions- relax, don't struggle
86   4

Freedom from self-will
87   2

God disciplines us
88   2

(Step 11)

Meditation and prayer
85   4

Morning prayer   86   3

Nightly prayer   86   2

Plans   86   3

Prayer and meditation
85   4

Pray- not selfishly
87   2

Prayer- thy will be done
88   1

Prayer- with wives
87   3

Self-will, pray for freedom
87   2

Undisciplined   88   2

Step 12   Description   59   3

Step 12 details   89   1

Alcoholics- carry the message
89   1

Alcoholics- sick people
90   1

Alcoholics- can't be persuaded
90   1

Carry the message to others
89   1

Cooperate, don't criticize
89   3

Helping others   89   1

Immunity through service
89   1

Service- helping others
89   1

Spouse   90   2

Service- immune from alcohol
89   1